Asian Detox Diet:

Cleansing the Body and Losing Weight the Asian Way

Disclaimer

Our ebooks are designed to provide information about the subject matter covered. They are sold with the understanding that the author and the publisher are not engaged in rendering legal, accounting, or other professional services. If legal advice or other professional assistance is required, the services of a competent professional person should be sought. Every effort has been made to make our ebooks as complete and accurate as possible. However, there may be mistakes both typographical and in content. Therefore, the texts should be used only as general guides and not as the ultimate sources of the subject matters covered. The authors and the publisher shall have neither liability nor responsibility to any person or entity with respect to any loss or damage caused or alleged to be caused directly or indirectly by the information covered in the ebooks.

Table of Contents

Introduction

People are always looking for ways to gain weight, lose weight, stay healthy, and so on. With so many different diets and exercise plans out there, it can be confusing to know which one is healthy and will work. The Asian detox diet is a healthy and safe way to keep the body clean from harmful chemicals and foods while maintaining a balanced nutritional plan.

Unlike most diet and detox plans, the Asian detox diet is an eating lifestyle that will keep the body clean and healthy. This book will give information on what is entailed in an Asian detox diet, precautions, food choices, and suggested recipes.

Many people make the mistake of eating nothing or eating very little when they diet. When the body feels itself starving, it naturally holds on to everything that is consumed, which is why people don't lose weight even though they aren't eating much. It's vital that any diet is balanced and contains sufficient nutrition to keep the body healthy.

Making good food choices is an important part of any diet. Simply eating less or purchasing prepared foods that advertise weight loss isn't enough. There are many tasty and healthy food choices that will leave a person fully satiated while having delicious meals.

Along with making these food choices, there are a large variety of spices and herbs that will make wonderfully flavorful meals while also keeping a person's food intake low and fulfilling. Understanding the types of foods that are healthy versus the foods that cause bad health is important when choosing a diet. The Asian detox diet is full of wonderful food and seasoning options that will make the diet enjoyable and a great lifestyle to which one can turn.

Understanding how to mix these foods and seasonings may be confusing. A few choice recipes will help give an idea how to prepare and mix delicious and healthy meals. There is no set rule of thumb for cooking Asian style except for keeping to fresh foods and seasonings, cooking with steam or heat versus fatty oils, and keeping to light and healthy meals.

The guidelines set forth in this book will hopefully help people find a more balanced way of eating while becoming healthier and happier.

Chapter 1: What are Detox Diets?

In the strictest sense, detoxification is when people are treated for addiction issues such as alcohol and drugs. People are admitted to a hospital in order to get medical treatment as they rid themselves of the addictive habit and to be monitored as their bodies adjust to having no chemicals inside them.

In a similar way, detox diets are a form of diet that people use to cleanse their bodies of toxins and harmful chemicals that build up, cause weight gain, and affect one's overall physical and mental health. There are many such diets and supplements to aid in body detox. The idea of cleansing the body goes back thousands of years in many religions in which fasting was a way of focusing the mind on more spiritual issues and ridding the body of unhealthy habits.

Nowadays, detox diets are a popular form of weight loss used by people around the world and seen in many news stories regarding celebrities. Some diets are liquid-only with seasonings and spices, others limit meat intake, and others are supplemented with expensive additives and tablets that must be purchased.

Regardless of what form of diet a person uses, care should be taken to maintain health and to refrain from depriving the body of the important nutrients it needs. Consulting a physician is important, particularly for a person who has health issues, is anemic, diabetic, or has any heart or lung condition.

Chapter 2: What is the Asian Detox Diet?

A look at the World Health Organization (WHO) website shows that the United States has one of the highest percentages of obesity, while Asian countries have about half the amount of obesity in their populations. The prevalence of fast food restaurants in the U.S. may be part of the issue. It's so easy to go through a drive-thru and pick up something quick to eat. Many families are busy and don't have the time to devote to cooking healthy meals. However, even with U.S. families who have home-cooked meals, a lot of the food is pre-packaged or processed. Many South American, Asian, and African countries have traditional family lifestyles, so cooking meals from natural products and from scratch are still the norm, thus allowing for healthier foods with less harmful ingredients.

The Asian detox diet originates with the Asian method of preparing and eating foods, most of which are natural and non-processed. Foods that go through processing plants tend to be injected with preservatives and fillers, which takes away from the purity and overall health of the product. Going back to organic and non-processed foods is a key concept in the Asian detox diet.

There are many vegetables, fruits, and spices that make the diet safe and flavorful. Most diets tend to be bland and boring, leaving the dieter unsatisfied and hungry. The Asian detox diet allows one to eat interesting foods with a variety of recipes and mixes that will make a person forget he or she is on a diet; however, it's not so much a diet as a lifestyle.

Meats are not a part of the detox diet, but with thought and research, certain meats such as fish products may be added to give protein. Many vegetarian diets have alternative sources of proteins. Also, carbonated drinks such as soda should be avoided. The high sodium in these drinks is not good for the body. Additionally, fruit juices that are not 100% or are from concentrate are avoided in the plan. Many of these beverages are high in sodium. Mixing and blending fruits is a favorable alternative in the diet.

Many of the ingredients are available at the grocery store. Others may need to be purchased from an Asian or international foods store. Items such as a blender and chopper might be handy to have around to prepare recipes.

Using methods of cooking such as steaming, boiling, or eating raw are the key to the success of the Asian detox diet. These simple methods of cooking leave out fat and allow food to be eaten in a more natural state.

The human body digests foods naturally, but when foods with unnatural ingredients and fillers are eaten on a regular basis, the body tends to get bloated, backed up, and has a hard time digesting the "garbage" sitting in the stomach and intestines. Roughage is an important dietary need that helps the body to do its job. When people neglect to eat foods such as fruits, vegetables, and healthy liquids, they are withholding an important digestive need from their system. Thus, they feel lethargic, tired, and heavy or bloated.

The Asian detox diet relies on roughage foods along with other natural items, bringing balance back to the body and allowing it to work properly. Using enemas as a way to empty the system is not safe. Eating the foods that will bring about natural elimination is safer and far easier.

Additionally, exercises such as walking, running, aerobics, and dance help with the body's circulation. The key to any diet is a mix of water, healthy foods, routine, and exercise. Starving the body simply depletes the blood, muscle, and tissue of much-needed nutrients to work properly. Plus, the body holds on to any food to make up for the starvation effect being forced onto it. It's vital that regular meals are eaten with moderation along with drinking non-soda beverages and getting proper exercise, even if it's only walking.

It's a fact that Asian countries tend to have lower rates of obesity, cancer, and heart disease than the United States, and their people tend to live longer lives. While there is no one actual Asian diet, there is a variety of foods that are available and can be fixed in a variety of ways. The central concept of the Asian detox diet is balance. Cooking at home using the Asian methods of eating will ensure a healthier lifestyle. An extra little tip is using pretty, smaller dishes when eating. The smaller plates will make the amounts appear larger and aesthetically appealing.

Chapter 3: Precautions

As with any diet, there are precautions that should be followed. The point of the detox diet is to help relieve the body of unwanted and unhealthy materials. The Asian detox diet is meant to be a way of eating healthy while getting proper exercise. There should be a variety of foods that will allow one to eat fully balanced meals while also getting the roughage and necessary foods that will keep the body cleansed.

If at any point, one notices feelings of lethargy, excessive tiredness, headaches, or general bad feelings, a doctor should be consulted. Many detox diets force people to only drink water with key spices and seasonings. This has caused many complications and even hospitalization. Any diet that denies the body healthy food and nutrients is harmful and should be avoided.

Detox diets are about ridding the body of unhealthy foods and chemicals. Weight loss should always happen slowly and naturally, coming from a consistent and healthy diet combined with exercise, proper sleep patterns, and avoidance of stress. The human body needs good bacteria to fight disease and bad toxins. If people are flushing the good bacteria out of their bodies, they are leaving themselves open to more health problems. Constant bowel movements also weaken the intestinal system and leave a person dehydrated.

The kidneys, liver, lungs, and skin are natural filters. Any detox diet should be short-term, no more than a week, and should be stopped if there are any negative side effects. Since many detox diets limit food intake, exercise is not possible due to the lack of energy. Additionally, dehydration is possible along with deficiency in vitamins and minerals that the body needs to function correctly. Muscles and tissue are also negatively affected if they are not receiving proper nutrition.

The Asian detox diet should be followed sensibly with regular and balanced meals. The whole point of the diet is that one is getting all the nutrients needed while keeping garbage foods out of the system. It is a more healthy way of detoxing on a continual basis while eating balanced meals and getting the proper nutrition.

It should be noted that when dining out, Asian restaurants are not cooking in the same manner as people cook in Asian countries. The food is Americanized and likely to contain many of the very foods that should be avoided.

Chapter 4: Foods that Work

Vegetables

Bamboo shoots are rich with nutrients, such as protein, and have been found to be helpful toward cancer prevention and weight loss.

Bean sprouts are rich with protein, along with vitamins A, B, C, D, E, and K, and minerals such as iron, potassium, calcium, phosphorous, magnesium and zinc. They also contain fiber, a key ingredient for the digestive cleansing system.

Bok choy is a cabbage type vegetable with green leaves. It is rich with vitamins A, C, and K, along with calcium, iron, potassium, and magnesium. It's been found to be helpful in preventing various cancers and helps reduce cholesterol.

Broccoli contains vitamins A, C, and K, as well as folate and potassium. It has also been found to be helpful in preventing colon and lung cancer.

Cabbage is a leafy vegetable that resembles iceberg lettuce. It contains vitamins C and K and is helpful for bone metabolism.

Carrots are an orange root vegetable that are rich in vitamins A and B and contain beta-carotenes. This vegetable is helpful for the health of the eyes, sperm reproduction, and helps to fight disease.

Chiles are small peppers that contain vitamins A and C, magnesium, and potassium.

Daikon radishes are long, white radishes rich in vitamin B-6 and C, and contain riboflavin, thiamin, iron, magnesium, copper, and calcium. They also have sulforaphane, which may aid against some cancers, and fiber, which helps in fighting colon cancer.

Eggplant is technically a fruit, but it is cooked as a vegetable. It contains potassium, folate, copper, magnesium, niacin, and fiber.

It's been found that those with kidney and gallbladder problems should avoid it.

Leeks are a type of onion, tubular in shape rather than round. They contain vitamins A, C, E, and K, folic acid, niacin, thiamin, riboflavin, copper, and iron. Leeks are helpful with keeping the blood vessels clear.

Lemons and limes are a citrus fruit that are strong in vitamin C and are helpful in fighting scurvy and infections. The citric acid helps digestion.

Lettuce has a variety of types from round to long leafy ones such as iceberg and romaine. Celtuce lettuce is a Chinese type of lettuce that is good for stir fries and stews. Lettuce contains vitamins A, K, and carotenes. It helps in bone metabolism.

Kale is a dark green leafy vegetable like lettuce that contains vitamins A, C, and K along with B-carotene, calcium, copper, iron, and manganese. It is helpful with eye retinal health, bones, and may aid in fighting Alzheimer's disease.

Mushrooms come in a variety of shapes, mostly whitish colors with roundish tops and stems. They contain vitamin D, which is good for bones. They also contain vitamin B2, biotin, and potassium. Mushrooms are a good gout reducer and an immune booster with antioxidants.

Mustard greens are spicy large, green, leafy plants that contain vitamins A, C, and K, calcium, iron, calcium, copper, manganese, and fiber. They help with mucus membranes, skin, and eyes. The fiber also helps control cholesterol levels.

Peppers are oblong-shaped, somewhat spicy vegetables that are hollow inside except for seeds and come in a variety of colors such as red, yellow, and green. They contain vitamins A and C and aid with collagen, blood vessels, organs, bones, and skin.

Pumpkins are large, round, orange gourds that contain vitamins A and C, copper, iron, and potassium. They are good for controlling cholesterol. Their seeds are also good for roasting and eating.

Scallions are smallish, long white onions with green tops that have vitamins A, C, and K, folates, and iron. They are good for helping to reduce blood pressure.

Seaweed is marine algae that have vitamins A and C, calcium, iron, fiber, and protein. Vitamin B12 makes seaweed a good choice for vegan diets. It aids in the digestive system. Buyers should beware of iodine levels in some products, and hijiki seaweed should not be consumed due to its levels of arsenic.

Snow peas are green pod vegetables of which the skin is eaten instead of shelled. They contain vitamins A, B6, C, and K, riboflavin, magnesium, phosphorous, fiber, potassium, thiamin, folate, iron, and manganese.

Spinach is a green leafy vegetable rich in iron and contains vitamins A, C, and K, copper, niacin, folates, thiamin, riboflavin, and fiber. Spinach is considered helpful in preventing prostate and colon cancer, and Alzheimer's. It is also helpful for red blood cells, mucus membranes, skin, and bones.

Sweet potatoes are root vegetables that are found in orange and deep purple colors. They contain vitamins A, B1, B2, B3, B6, and C, manganese, copper, pantothenic acids, biotin, potassium, and fiber. They are a good alternative for diabetics and aid in the digestive system. Sweet potatoes also contain antioxidants and anti-inflammatory agents.

Taro root is an oblong root vegetable with large leafy tops. The root contains vitamin E, fiber, copper, and potassium. It's similar to a potato and contains healthy carbohydrates.

Turnips are round root vegetables with a white and purple coloring. They contain vitamin C and have been found to be helpful in preventing cancers and inflammation, and they aid in boosting the body's immunity.

Water chestnuts (Chinese) are a roundish vegetable with a brown outside and white inside. Buyers should beware of purchasing the thorny European water chestnuts as they contain toxins. Chinese water chestnuts maintain a crunchy texture even after cooking and contain vitamin B6, copper, potassium, riboflavin, and manganese. They have various benefits depending on how prepared, such as aiding in nausea, jaundice, and detoxification when juiced. They're helpful with inflammation when the powder is turned into a paste, and work as a cough elixir when mixed with water. The inside contains puchin, which is an antibiotic.

Fruits

Apricots are a small, round bright orange fruit with a velvety skin. They contain vitamins A and C, fiber, potassium, and copper. They are helpful in preventing heart disease, inflammation, and also help the eyes and the digestive system.

Bananas are long, curved white fruit with a yellow skin that's peeled. They contain vitamins A, B6, and C, fiber, and potassium. Bananas are good for the heart and reduce blood pressure, aid in preventing depression, help muscle relaxation, and aid in the bones' absorption of calcium.

Cherries are small, round bright red drupe or stone fruit that contain vitamins A and C, copper, and potassium. Cherries may be helpful in relieving gout arthritis, fibromyalgia, and sports injuries. Their antioxidants help in preventing various cancers, soothe brain neurons, and aid in reducing blood pressure.

Coconuts are round, tough fruits with a hard shell yet hollow inside with a white meaty substance and a tasty juice. Its meat is higher in fat but helpful in bringing healthy cholesterol into the system. Coconut milk is good for cooking in place of oils. Coconut contains vitamin C, thiamin, copper, iron, manganese, phosphorous, and selenium. The fruit is helpful in anti-aging, digestion, and metabolism.

Dates are grape-like fruit that grow in bunches on trees and are treated like raisins for eating. They contain fiber, niacin, pantothenic acid, pyridoxine, riboflavin, thiamin, vitamin A, potassium, calcium, copper, iron, magnesium, manganese, phosphorous, and zinc. They are easy to digest and help renew energy, so are a popular addition to fasting cultures. The fiber helps in the digestive system and aid in preventing colon, prostate, breast, lung, and pancreatic cancers. Dates are also useful for their anti-inflammatory and anti-hemorrhaging properties. They may also aid in blood pressure and heart health.

Dragon fruit are small, cactus fruit with a pinkish outside and a white inside. The flesh and seeds are both edible, having a sweet, crunchy texture. They're good for eating fresh or pureed into smoothies. They contain fiber, thiamin, riboflavin, and iron and are a good source of vitamin C. Dragon fruit help the immune system and aid the body's ability to get rid of toxins, which helps the cells heal. The seeds are good for relieving constipation.

Grapes are small round fruit that grow in bunches, available in green, red, and blue/black varieties. They contain vitamins C and K, pyridoxine, riboflavin, thiamin, copper, and iron. Grapes are rich in resveratrol, an antioxidant that aids in fighting cancer, Alzheimer's, heart disease, and degenerative nerve disease. It also helps reduce the risk of stroke.

Kiwi fruit, or Chinese gooseberry, grow on large woody vines and have a brown, hairy skin with a seedy, green fruit inside. They contain fiber, folates, vitamins A, E, K, potassium, calcium, copper, iron, magnesium, manganese, and zinc. They're especially rich in vitamin C. Kiwi are a little more heavy in calories, but their health benefits outweigh this fact. They aid in protecting the colon mucus membrane, are a strong antioxidant that fight infections, and help in bone mass. They have also been helpful in preventing Alzheimer's and aid in keeping the blood vessels healthy.

Longan is also known as dragon eye due to the large pit inside its fruit interior. Longans are round and covered in a brown skin. They can be eaten raw, dried, or frozen for later. They contain vitamin C, thiamin, riboflavin, iron, potassium, magnesium, and zinc. They have an antioxidant that helps fight heart disease, chronic inflammation, and some cancers. They also aid in the cardiovascular system, improve energy, and bring better health to the skin.

Lychee is a pulpy fruit covered with a bumpy brown skin that contains vitamin C, folates, niacin, pyridoxine, riboflavin, potassium, copper, magnesium, manganese, and phosphorous. The seeds should not be eaten. The fruit has been found to contain oligonol, which works as an antioxidant and anti-influenza agent and helps in blood circulation, reduces weight, and protects the skin. The high rate of vitamin C aids in fighting infections. Lychees are also good for improving metabolism, controlling the heart rate, and producing red blood cells.

Mandarins (also known as tangerines) are related to oranges but are smaller, have thinner skins that are easier to peel, and are sweeter. They contain fiber, folates, niacin, pantothenic acid, pyridoxine, riboflavin, thiamin, vitamins A and C, potassium, calcium, copper, iron, and magnesium. They are a good antioxidant, aiding in collagen synthesis, the healing of wounds, fight viruses and cancer, and help in preventing cholesterol buildup as helping in regular bowel movements.

Mangoes are a fleshy, roundish fruit that come in varieties of yellow, red, or orange-red. They contain carbohydrates, fiber, folates, niacin, pyridoxine, riboflavin, thiamin, vitamins C, A, E, and K, potassium, copper, iron, and magnesium. Studies show they may aid in fighting colon, breast, and prostate cancers, as well as leukemia. Mangoes are also good for vision, healthy mucus membranes, skin, and can help control the heart rate and blood pressure.

Melon is also known as cantaloupe; it has a tannish, roughly textured skin with a fleshy fruit inside, with seeds in the center. Melons contain carbohydrates, fiber, folates, niacin, pyridoxine, riboflavin, thiamin, vitamins A, C, E, and K, potassium, calcium, copper, iron, magnesium, manganese, and zinc. The high amount of vitamin A makes them a good choice to aid in vision, mucus membranes, and skin health. The antioxidants are good for fighting various cancers, and there are also nutrients that help control the heart rate and blood pressure. High amounts of vitamin C also make melons a good source of protection against infections and viruses.

Oranges are a citrus fruit with an orange skin and pulpy fruit inside. They contain protein, fiber, folates, niacin, pantothenic acid, pyridoxine, riboflavin, thiamin, vitamins A, C, E, and K, potassium, calcium, copper, iron, magnesium, manganese, and zinc. Oranges are a wonderful source of energy, a great thirst-quencher, and easy to carry. Their pectin is useful for reducing cholesterol; the large amount of vitamin C makes them a great antioxidant and help in fighting infections and inflammations. They also help keep skin glowing, help the vision, and keep mucus membranes healthy. Blood pressure is also aided with the nutrients in oranges.

Papaya is an oval, rounded fruit with a greenish-yellow outside and orange fleshy inside, with black beaded seeds. It contains fiber, folates, niacin, pantothenic acid, pyridoxine, riboflavin, thiamin, vitamins A, C, E, and K, potassium, calcium, iron, magnesium, and phosphorous. Papaya helps maintain regular bowel movements and has a high amount of vitamin C to help the immune system and fight infections. It is also good for keeping mucus membranes healthy, keeps skin healthy, and may aid in the prevention of cancer. The B vitamins help metabolism, and potassium is good for helping keep the heart rate and blood pressure controlled.

Pears are a bell-shaped fruit available in a couple varieties, such as the Asian and European pear. The Asian are rather crisp whereas the European pear is more soft and juicy when ripe. There are yellow, green, and red-orange varieties with white insides. They contain fiber, folates, niacin, pantothenic acid, pyridoxine, riboflavin, thiamin, vitamins A, C, E, and K, potassium, copper, iron, magnesium, manganese, phosphorous, and zinc. They're helpful in avoiding colon cancer and help reduce cholesterol. Pears have been found to be the least allergenic, so are popular for those with allergies and may be found in medicines to help treat colitis, gallbladder issues, arthritis, and gout.

Pineapple has a cylindrical shape, with sharp layers of husk on the outside, and a juicy, sweet fruit inside. Pineapple contains fiber, folates, niacin, pyridoxine, riboflavin, thiamin, vitamins A, C, E, and K, potassium, calcium, copper, iron, magnesium, manganese, and phosphorous. Pectin makes it a good digestive aid; it also has properties that help with anti-clotting and fighting cancer. It has been shown to help reduce arthritis, indigestion, and worm infestation. It's a great antioxidant, fighting infections and boosting immunity. Pineapple helps give healthy mucus membranes, skin, and eyes. It also helps with controlling blood pressure and the heart rate, as well as aiding in red blood cell synthesis.

Grains

Barley is a type of grass used to make cereal. It's a good alternative for diabetics. Its fiber helps maintain good bowel movements. It contains niacin, thiamin, selenium, iron, magnesium, zinc, phosphorous, and copper. It's cholesterol-free. It also has antioxidants and may aid in reducing heart disease, diabetes, and cancer.

Buckwheat is not a cereal grain or wheat; it's a green, leafy plant with flowers and is treated like grain. Buckwheat contains carbohydrates, protein, fat, fiber, folates, niacin, pantothenic acid, riboflavin, thiamin, potassium, calcium, copper, iron, magnesium, manganese, phosphorous, selenium, zinc, and various amino acids. The fiber content helps with the digestive system; it's gluten free. Buckwheat helps reduce inflammation, and its antioxidant properties are good for the blood vessels. It also helps with red blood cells and may aid in depression and headache.

Noodles:

- Soba noodles are made with buckwheat and resemble spaghetti but have a nuttier flavor. They're a good source of fiber and have similar health benefits to buckwheat.

- Rice is a grain with no fats, sodium, or cholesterol. Brown rice is higher in phosphorous, fiber, protein, and potassium than white rice. Both contain carbohydrates, protein, calcium, thiamin, and niacin.

Nuts, Seeds, and Legumes

Almonds are a nut that grown on a tree similar to peaches. They grow inside a peach-like fruit, which breaks open upon ripening to reveal the small almond in its brown shell. Almonds contain protein, fat, fiber, folates, niacin, pantothenic acid, pyridoxine, riboflavin, thiamin, vitamin E, potassium, calcium, copper, iron, magnesium, manganese, phosphorous, selenium, and zinc. The fats in almond are good for lowering bad cholesterol and raising good cholesterol. They also act as an antioxidant, maintaining mucus membranes and skin. Since almonds don't contain gluten protein, they are a good alternative for people with allergies. All the B vitamins aid in cell metabolism. Almond oil is also a good emollient and can be used for cooking.

Beans

- Adzuki is a red-brown bean with a sweet and nutty taste, frequently used in Japanese desserts. Adzuki beans contain carbohydrates, protein, iron, potassium, and folic acid.

- Edamame is boiled green soybeans and make a good snacking food. They contain fiber, polyunsaturated fat, monounsaturated fat, protein, carbohydrate, sodium, vitamins A and C, iron, and calcium.

- Mung beans are pea-like beans that grow inside long, black pods. They contain vitamins A, B, C, and E, calcium, iron, magnesium, fiber, and potassium. They aid in reducing heart disease and risk of breast cancer. They are good for diabetics, reduce cholesterol levels, and help the liver and skin.

- Soybeans are a whitish bean encased in pods. There is some controversy as to their overall health benefits, with some concern over their working against nutrients and possible side effects such as allergies and issues in reproductive systems. They contain fiber, saturated fats, vitamin C, calcium, and iron. They are used in a variety of products, such as soy milk, tofu, and soy nuts.

Cashews are the "clapper" of a bell-like apple, which is an extremely juicy fruit. The cashew nut is encased in a highly acidic shell that must be burned before opening so as to avoid skin burns. Cashews contain carbohydrates, protein, fat, fiber, folates, niacin, pantothenic acid, pyridoxine, riboflavin, thiamin, vitamins C, E, and K, sodium, potassium, calcium, copper, iron, magnesium, manganese, phosphorous, selenium, and zinc. Although high in calories, they are full of good nutrients to help fight disease and cancer. Their fatty content aids in reducing bad cholesterol while raising good cholesterol and helps the heart.

Hazelnuts grow on a flowering tree and are the kernel within a rounded pod. They contain carbohydrates, protein, fat, fiber, folates, niacin, pantothenic acid, pyridoxine, riboflavin, thiamin, vitamins C, E, and K, potassium, calcium, copper, iron, magnesium, manganese, phosphorous, and zinc. Hazelnuts lower bad cholesterol while raising good cholesterol and aid in preventing coronary artery disease and strokes. They also help in preventing diseases and cancers. Hazelnuts are good for expectant mothers as they help prevent anemia and aid in preventing neural tube defects in babies. The vitamin E protects cell membrane, mucus membranes, and help skin. The nut is also gluten free and good for people with wheat allergies or diabetes.

Lentils are beans that grow in small pods. Like other beans, they are a good source of fiber and protein. They also contain folate, iron, and B6. Lentils help cell growth and immunity, aid in preventing breast cancer, and are a protection against artery disease and birth defects. They come in a variety of types and colors and are a good alternative for vegans.

Miso is a fermented paste, usually consisting of soybeans, that has a salty taste. Miso is commonly mixed with brown rice, white rice, barley, ginger, or buckwheat. It contains vitamins B2, E, and K, calcium, iron, potassium, choline, lecithin, fiber, and protein. It is good for lowering bad cholesterol, keeps skin healthy, aids in the digestive system, and also strengthens the immune system. Miso is good for those with diabetes and may reduce chances of cancer, cardiovascular disease, and aging.

Sesame seeds grow in small pods on flowering, leafy plants. They contain carbohydrates, protein, fat, fiber, folates, niacin, pyridoxine, riboflavin, thiamin, vitamin E, potassium, calcium, copper, iron, magnesium, manganese, phosphorous, selenium, and zinc. Sesame seeds are a source of energy, act as an antioxidant, can prevent birth defects, and reduce anxiety and neurosis. They are also good for bone mineralization, red blood cell production, and aid in cardiac and skeletal muscle action.

Tofu is soymilk that has been coagulated and pressed into curds. Tofu contains protein, fat, calcium, and iron. It is used in place of meat in stir fries, salads, and soups.

Tempeh is another soy product that is fermented and pressed into cake form. It is used in stews, soups, and kebabs.

Herbs and Spices

Amchoor is made from unripe green mangoes. It is a powder that has a tart taste and used for acidity. Lime or lemon juice can be substituted.

Asafetida is a large fennel-like plant. Its gum resin is powdered and has a strong onion-like flavor. It should be used sparingly due to its strong flavor. Garlic or onion powder may be substituted.

Basil is a green herb that has a slightly sweet flavor to it and blends well in tomato dishes, salads, soups, and sauces. Fresh basil is easy to grow at home.

Cardamom is a spice that is best used straight from the pod. There are green, black, and Madagascar cardamom, but green is the most popular. In its powdered form, it loses much of its flavor. It has a spicy-sweet taste. Cardamom is used in curries and lentil dishes and goes well with coffee, oranges, peace, rice, and squash.

Chiles are hot peppers that go well with many dishes, adding spice and flavor.

Cloves are aromatic, unopened pink flower buds of the evergreen clove tree, which are picked and then dried. They have a warm, sweet taste that go well with ginger, pumpkin, split pea and bean soups, baked beans, and chili.

Coriander is the seed of cilantro plants. It has a sweet, slightly lemony flavor and is good in chili and curry dishes.

Curry leaves are not to be confused with curry powder. They are an edible herb that add a subtle aroma to dishes and complement spiced foods. They can be grown at home and freeze well. They have no flavor once powdered.

Fennel is a bulbous plant with multiple stalks like celery that are cut off. It's a good vegetable for using like celery or cooking. It can also be used with ginger to make a good tea to aid digestion.

Fenugreek is a bitter herb that's used in curries, vegetables, and lentil dishes. Pregnant women should be careful as large quantities may induce labor. Fenugreek comes in many forms and has medicinal uses, as well.

Garlic is an onion type of vegetable that has a strong flavor. It can be roasted, boiled, or eaten raw.

Ginger is a flowering root plant that can be used in its fresh tubular form, minced, or powdered. It has a light spicy, tangy, warm sweet flavor that goes well in many dishes, particularly with fruits or vegetables.

Ginseng is the root of a flowering plant. It lasts a long time when dehydrated. Ginseng has a lot of health properties and can be used in soups and beverages, as well as food dishes. However, ginseng may have negative effects on children and pregnant or breastfeeding women, so care should be taken and a doctor consulted. It should also not be overused.

Kaffir lime leaves are the dark, glossy green leaves found on the kaffir lime, a round and knobby fruit. They add a distinctive lime-lemon flavor to dishes such as soups, stews, salads, and curries.

Masala is an Arabic word meaning "seasonings." The most popular is garam masala, which goes well with onion-based sauces. Chaat masala is tart and salty, while chai masala is good in hot teas.

Mint is a leafy plant that can be grown at home. It has a fairly strong flavor and fragrance and adds a cool taste to sweet, savory recipes.

Parsley is a leafy herb that has a strong flavor and can be grown at home. It is usually used as a garnish but adds flavor to salads, sauces, marinades, and soups.

Pepper (black) comes from peppercorns, which grow on leafy plants. Fresh ground peppercorn is best. It's a versatile spice that adds flavor to any dish.

Star anise is a star-shaped dark brown pod with small seeds within and grown on small evergreen trees. It has a more bitter taste than regular anise and gives a licorice flavor to dishes. It goes well with fish, leeks, pears, pumpkin, shrimp, and poultry.

Turmeric comes from a reddish-orange root related to the ginger family. It has a peppery, warm, bitter taste with a mild aroma. It goes well in curries and soups, and adds flavor to cauliflower, broccoli, and onions.

Wasabi is a leafy plant related to cabbage, horseradish, and mustard. The root is grated and used in seasoning food. The leaves may also be used in recipes. Many American restaurants do not serve real wasabi, but instead serve a horseradish substitute.

Beverages

Teas are a natural complement to meals. Popular blends include oolong, orange pekoe, ginseng, and chai.

Water is an important supplement to any diet.

Coconut milk is a flavorful and healthy alternative to sodas.

Fruit juices made from fresh fruit are a healthy and delicious choice. Several types of fruit can be blended, giving variety.

Soy milk is a good alternative to milk products and can be found in various flavors.

Chapter 5: Foods to Avoid

Red meats such as beef products (hamburger, stew beef, steak, etc.) and pork (pork chops, sausage, bacon, etc.) should be avoided. These all contain high-cholesterol and fatty ingredients that can cause over-weight issues and clog the arteries.

Carbohydrates, such as breads, rolls, buns, white rice (in excess), pasta, and donuts, pastries, and cakes, are all full of sugars and should be avoided.

Dairy products such as milk, cheese, coffee creamer, butter, and mayonnaise are all rich in fatty contents.

Condiments such as ketchup, mustard, jellies and jams, syrups, and so on are full of additives, preservatives, salt, and sugars.

Pre-packaged foods such as boxed mixes, frozen meals, canned products such as soups, pastes, and broths contain a vast amount of preservatives and additives, salts, and sugars.

Carbonated drinks, canned juice drinks (unless from concentrate and 100% with no additives), pre-mixed teas, hot chocolate, and other pre-packaged or prepared drinks should all be off the diet due to their high content of sodium, sugars, and other additives.

Fast food products such as hamburgers, chicken products, French fries, sodas, pies, and so on are all full of fillers, additives, carbohydrates, salt, fats, and sugar. They are the main cause of health issues and the need for cleansing of the body. The fatty substances and high amounts of sugars and salt all cause problems within the body and are a direct link to obesity, especially on a regular basis. Beware of the advertising for healthy choices, as most prepared foods still contain preservatives and additives that are not good for the body.

The purpose of the Asian detox diet is to cleanse the system and clean out the bad ingredients that make one feel lethargic, heavy, bloated, and run down. For a true detox cleansing, all meat should be avoided for a week or so, and the diet should focus on fresh vegetables, fruits, liquids, and purity of meals. After about a week of this pure diet, fish and poultry can be introduced into the diet to ensure a balanced diet of proteins with the fruit and vegetables, grains, and dairy products. It is recommended that red meat is only used once a month. Exercise is also an important aspect of a balanced diet.

Chapter 6: Recipes

Red Curry with Vegetables

1 pound sweet potato, cut into 1-inch cubes

1 14-ounce can light coconut milk (100%)

½ cup water

1-2 tsp red Thai curry paste

½ pound green beans (trimmed and cut into 1-inch pieces)

1 tbsp brown sugar

2 teaspoons lime juice (100% natural or fresh limes)

¼ tsp salt

1/3 cup chopped fresh cilantro

1 lime, quartered

Mix coconut milk, water, and curry paste. Stir well and add sweet potato. Bring to a boil. Reduce to a simmer and cook covered, stirring occasionally, until the sweet potato is barely tender (four minutes or so). Add the green beans and brown sugar, returning to a simmer and cook covered, stirring occasionally, under the beans are tender-crisp (two to four minutes). Stir in lime juice and salt. Sprinkle with cilantro and serve with lime wedges.

Note: Water can be replaced with chicken broth from freshly boiled chicken breast

Tropical Cucumber Salad

1 tsp freshly grated lime zest

2 tbsp lime juice

2 tsp light brown sugar – can be omitted and 1 tsp honey used instead

1 tsp rice vinegar

¼ tsp crushed red pepper

1 medium cucumber, diced

1 avocado, diced

1 mango, diced

¼ cup chopped, fresh cilantro

Mix all the juices and spices together, whisking until blended well. Add in the cucumber, avocado, mango, and cilantro. Toss gently to mix.

Korean Tofu Soup

8 cups broth from freshly boiled chicken (or substitute with coconut water)

2 tbsp finely chopped garlic

2 tbsp finely grated fresh ginger

½ cup uncooked brown rice

½ tsp salt

1 tsp toasted sesame oil

1-2 tsp hot chiles paste or minced chiles

2 scallions, finely chopped

1 tbsp sesame seeds

1 cup tofu (substituted for chicken)

Combine broth or coconut water, garlic and ginger in a Dutch oven; bring to a boil. Add rice, reduce heat to a medium boil and simmer for 12 to 15 minutes. Stir in salt, sesame oil, and chiles to taste. Add tofu and heat through. Garnish with scallions and sesame seeds.

Sweet and Sour Tofu

One half of a fresh pineapple, diced (preserve the juice to be used, approx. ¼ cup)

3 tbsp rice-wine vinegar

2 tbsp reduced-sodium soy sauce

½ tsp honey

2 tbsp coconut oil, split

14 ounces of extra-firm, water-packed tofu, drained and diced

2 tsp cornstarch

2 tbsp minced garlic

1 tbsp minced ginger

1 large red bell pepper, sliced into strips

1 large green bell pepper, sliced into strips

1. Whisk pineapple juice, vinegar, soy sauce, and honey in a medium bowl until smooth. Place tofu in a large bowl and mix with 3 tbsp of the sauce; marinade for 5 – 30 minutes.

2. Add cornstarch to the remaining sauce and whisk well.

3. Heat 1 tbsp coconut oil in a medium, non-stick pan over medium heat; add marinated tofu to the pan once hot; use a slotted spoon and add leftover marinade to the remaining sauce. Cook the tofu 7 – 9 minutes, stirring often. Remove and keep to the side.

4. Add remaining coconut oil to the pan, heat over medium heat. Add the garlic and ginger; stir while cooking for about 30 seconds. Add the red and green peppers; cook while stirring constantly until tender, about 2 – 3 minutes. Pour in the reserved sauce and cook, stirring until thickened, about 30 seconds. Add the tofu and pineapple, stirring gently until heated through, about 2 minutes.

Quick Kimchi

1 small head napa (Chinese) cabbage, cored and diced

2 cloves garlic, minced

¼ cup water

2 tbsp distilled white vinegar

1 tbsp toasted sesame oil

2 tsp fresh ginger, finely grated

¾ tsp salt

¼ tsp honey

½ tsp crushed red pepper

3 scallions, diced

1 carrot, peeled and grated

1. Combine cabbage, garlic, and water in a large saucepan; bring to a boil over high heat. Reduce heat to medium-low and cook, stirring once or twice until tender, about 4 – 5 minutes.
2. Meanwhile, whisk vinegar, oil, ginger, honey, and crushed red pepper in a large bowl.
3. Add the cabbage, scallions, and carrot to the bowl and toss to combine. Refrigerate about 25 minutes before serving.

Coconut-Lime Chicken and Snow Peas

1 cup coconut milk

¼ cup lime juice

2 tbsp brown sugar

½ tsp salt

4 ounces chicken breasts, sliced into strips

4 cups shredded romaine lettuce

1 cup shredded red cabbage

1 cup sliced snow peas

3 tbsp minced fresh cilantro

2 tbsp minced red onion

1. Preheat oven to 400F degrees. Whisk coconut milk, lime juice, sugar and salt in an 8-by-8 inch glass baking dish. Transfer ¼ cup of the dressing to a large bowl; set aside. Place chicken in the baking dish; bake until cooked through, about 20 minutes.

2. Meanwhile, add lettuce, cabbage, snow peas, cilantro, and onion to the large bowl with the dressing; toss to coat. Split onto two plates.

3. Transfer the chicken to a cutting board and slice into thin strips. Arrange the chicken on the salads. Drizzle 1 tsp of the coconut cooking sauce over each plated salad.

Conclusion

Eating balanced meals, exercising, and refraining from unhealthy food choices will all work together with the Asian detox diet to give a person a lot of energy, balance, and good health overall. Once one has gotten adjusted to buying and preparing natural healthy foods, it won't feel like a diet at all, but a positive way of staying healthy and balanced.

Planning ahead and writing down meal plans will make shopping easier and less expensive. It will also help make it easier to maintain the diet. If the needed foods aren't available at meal time, it may be easier to slip and make unhealthy choices as a matter of convenience.

Once one has adjusted and gotten used to cooking in a healthier manner, it will be easy to maintain the lifestyle and stay healthy. As stated, the Asian detox diet is not a diet so much as a lifestyle. Many people find that once they go off a diet, they put on the lost weight with additional pounds added. By making this diet a way of life, there will be no fear of gaining back unwanted weight or losing the healthy feelings.

While the Asian detox diet calls for no meat, once one has cleansed the body of the bad fillers, fats, and bloated feelings, it is easy to add fish, chicken, and eggs to gain more choices and make one feel as if he or she is coming off a diet. These meats are all healthier than red meat and can add more flavor and texture to the meals. It is recommended that red meat only be consumed once a month.

Finally, maintaining a positive attitude, relieving stress, and getting regular exercise while eating healthy all work side-by-side to ensure a healthy, happy, and balanced life. No diet works if a person is allowing life to keep the mental mind as unbalanced as the body. Life is full of stress. Eating healthy and maintaining a balanced routine may leave one feeling less stressed than ever thought possible.

Stay healthy and enjoy!

If you enjoyed this book please consider purchasing and reading:

Asians Don't Diet: The Food and Lifestyle of Asians to Live a Long and Healthy Life

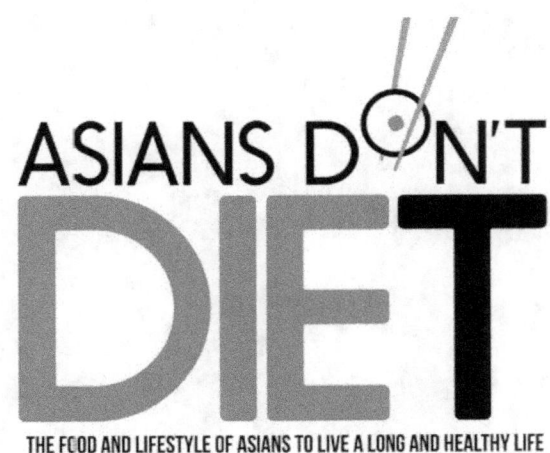